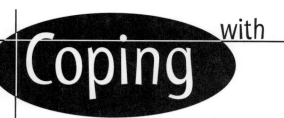

STUTTERING

Melanie Ann Apel

THE ROSEN PUBLISHING GROUP, INC./NEW YORK

Published in 2000 by The Rosen Publishing Group, Inc.
29 East 21st Street, New York, NY 10010

First Edition

Cover Photo by Shalhevet Moshe

Library of Congress Cataloging-in-Publication Data

Apel, Melanie Ann.
      Coping with stuttering / Melanie Ann Apel
            p.   cm. — (Coping)
      Includes bibliographical references and index.
      Summary: Discusses the causes of the speech disorder, stuttering,
explains how to cope in situations with family and friends as well as at
school, and tells where to get help.
      ISBN 0-8239-2970-1 (library binding)
      1. Stuttering Juvenile literature. 2. Stuttering in children Juvenile
literature.   [1. Stuttering.] I. Title. II. Series: Coping with series
(New York, N.Y.)
RC424.A626 2000
616.85'54—dc21   99-38580
                                                                              CIP

About the Author

Melanie Ann Apel is a pediatric respiratory therapist at Children's Memorial Hospital in Chicago, Illinois. She has a bachelor's degree in respiratory care and another in theater arts. Melanie has written six children's books on health-related topics, and she is currently working on another six. She is also working on two books about cystic fibrosis. Melanie lives in Glenview, Illinois.

Contents

Introduction

Ben sat by the phone with Grace's phone number written on a piece of paper in front of him.

"Just call her, man," said Doug. "Just pick up the phone and call her, and when she answers ask her out."

"Bu-bu-bu-but what if I start to sssstutter?" Ben asked with exasperation.

"You won't. Listen, man, just relax and take it easy. Go slow," Doug suggested.

"You just don't und-d-d-derstand!" said Ben. "It's n-n-not that easy! Besides, your t-t-telling me to calm down makes it wwwworse."

"Ben, just call her."

"OK," Ben said. He picked up the phone and dialed the number in front of him. After two rings he heard "Hello!" He recognized Grace's pretty voice. He smiled and opened his mouth to return the greeting, but nothing came out!

"Hello?" Grace said again.

Ben tried again, but still the words seemed to get stuck inside his mouth.

"Hello! Is anyone there?" Grace demanded.

Finally Ben started, "H-h-h—"

But by then Grace said, "Creep!" and hung up.

Ben put the phone down. "Sssee? I t-t-told you," he said.

"I'm sorry, man. Do you want me to call her back and ask her out for you?" Doug suggested. Ben told Doug that he didn't think Grace would be interested in going out with a guy who stuttered so badly that he couldn't even call her and ask her out himself. Doug didn't know what to tell his friend because he was afraid there was a chance that Ben was right. Maybe Grace wouldn't want to go out with Ben.

You stutter. It's no secret, or maybe it is because you have become really good at hiding your stuttering from other people. How do you feel about the fact that you stutter? Does it embarrass you or make you angry? Do you pretend to be shy so that you do not have to speak to other people? Maybe you really do not care that you stutter. If you are reading this book, however, chances are you are at least somewhat bothered by your stuttering. You are a teenager now, and you probably have figured out that you are not going to outgrow your stutter. But you probably hoped that you would, didn't you?

Being a teenager is not easy. You have so many things to worry about—school, friends, family, grades, dating, being popular, getting into college, fighting acne, what your hair looks like, whether you are tall enough or short enough or thin enough, and so on. On top of all this, you have to worry about stuttering. This is most likely one of your biggest worries at this point. You may be afraid that stuttering is going to get in the way of having a fun high school experience, dating, getting into a good college, or even getting a job. Stuttering is probably the one thing about yourself that you wish you could change more than anything else. Well, here is something that you will be very happy to know: Stuttering does not have to be a handicap, nor does it have to keep you from enjoying life. You can overcome your stuttering!

Believe it or not, many people who stutter have led amazing lives. Famous actors, television personalities, professional athletes, best-selling authors, businessmen, and even kings have been stutterers! You probably know the names of many of these famous people, yet you would be quite surprised to learn that they are in fact stutterers. Have you heard of the actor James Earl Jones or television journalist John Stossel? What about the legendary Marilyn Monroe? Did you know that all of these people had to overcome a stutter? So did singers Robert Merrill and Carly Simon. Perhaps you thought that stutterers could only be people who stay at home and do not work, or who only do work that does not involve verbal communication with other people. If you thought any of those things, you were wrong. A person who stutters can be whatever he or she wants to be. It may just require a little more time and effort, and it may certainly take an extra bit of courage, but you can do it! You have already made a very important first step by starting to read this book. What you have to do now is take control of your stuttering rather than letting it have control over you. You are in charge now. It is up to you to learn all you can about stuttering and to get yourself some help. This book will tell you all about how to do just that. So if you are ready to help yourself, get comfortable and read on!

Stuttering:
A Speech Disorder

Stuttering is a speech disorder that affects over three million Americans. That is about 5 percent of the population, or five out of every 100 people. If that does not sound like a lot of stutterers, consider that five out of every 100 people is the same ratio as one out of every twenty people. Now doesn't that seem like quite a lot of stutterers? If you are that one person in twenty, you now may realize that stuttering is fairly common and that you are certainly not alone. If you are male, you are even more likely to be a stutterer because four times as many males stutter as females. You also may be surprised to learn that people in all parts of the world, speaking different languages, stutter. Four percent of the world's children stutter. Most stuttering begins when children are three or four years old. Almost all stutterers are diagnosed by the time they are seven years old. About half of children who stutter when they are very young outgrow their stuttering before they are teenagers, but the other half enter adulthood still stuttering.

People who stutter are just as smart, just as normal, and certainly just as well adjusted as people who are not stutterers. However, stutterers are usually very self-conscious about the fact that they stutter. Some are so self-conscious about their stuttering that they avoid social situations, dating, parties, answering questions in class, talking on the tele-phone, speaking in public, and even going for the job or career they really want. None of this makes a stutterer any less intelligent or less able to do a job than a person who does not stutter. It means only that the stutterer has more to overcome when he or she is in a social or work situation.

People who stutter can get help for their problem. Specialists, called speech therapists or speech patholo-gists, can help stutterers work toward fluent speech. Speech therapy takes time. No cure for stuttering exists, but a stutterer definitely can be helped. With hard work, persistence, time, and patience, people who stutter can achieve speech that they can be proud of.

In the chapters that follow, you will learn exactly what stuttering is, why you stutter, and how you can over-come your stuttering so that you can feel free to live the life you have always dreamed of. You will learn what you need to know about getting help for your stuttering. If you are not a person who stutters but know someone who is, you will find it very helpful to read the sections on how to help a stutterer. At the back of the book is a list of further reading and resources so that you will know where to go to read more about stuttering and how to get professional help.

The Causes of Stuttering

Doctors believe that stuttering comes from a combination of hereditary and environmental factors. This means that if you stutter, it may be because of the family you were born into and the people and situations around you.

Researchers have not yet been able to prove that stuttering is genetically inherited, but they do know that there is a tendency for stuttering to run in families. The actual stuttering may not be an inherited trait, but a susceptibility to becoming a stutterer may be inherited.

If you are a stutterer, perhaps you have an older brother who stutters or an uncle who is a mild stutterer. Twins have been studied to see whether or not there is a genetic predisposition to stuttering. With identical twins, who share the same DNA, it was found that if one stutters there is a much greater chance that the other twin will stutter as well. With fraternal twins, however, who are produced from separate eggs and share only similar DNA, much less of a chance exists that both twins will stutter. Female stutterers are more likely to have children who stutter. Of course, some stutterers just stutter all by themselves; that is, there is no family history of stuttering at all. Doctors do not know why these patterns exist, but when there are stutterers in a family, it is important to keep an eye on the speech patterns of all the children as they are learning to speak. Identifying a child as a stutterer at a very young age is a great help, because the earlier the child begins speech therapy, the better off he or she will be as an adult. Studies have shown that if children identified as potential stutterers receive therapy at an early age, many will not become stutterers. The complicated relationship that researchers see between biological and social factors is part of what makes it so hard to discover the causes of stuttering.

Another more obvious cause of stuttering is brain injury. If a person has had a serious accident and suffered head trauma, for example, this could cause a nonstutterer to become a stutterer. By now you most likely know whether or not you have suffered some type of brain injury, whether someone else in your family stutters, or whether you are the only stutterer you know among your relatives. It is not really necessary for you to know exactly what causes you to stutter. The reason for your stutter makes little difference in terms of your therapy. What matters is working to control and correct it. You can get help for your stuttering and learn to speak clearly, easily, comfortably, and fluently.

One thing to keep in mind is that there is a difference between actual stuttering and simple speech disfluency. Most children and even some teenagers and adults stutter a little bit at times or experience mild speech disfluencies once in a while. Children between the ages of two and five actually may seem to stutter quite a bit, but they really are just experiencing the normal speech disfluencies of children learning to speak. For most children, once they pass through these years of intense language development, their stuttering or disfluency gradually tapers off until it is completely gone. However, if you are a stutterer now as a teenager, you did not pass through this stage so easily. A child is best off if he or she starts a speech therapy program right away when it appears that the normal speech disfluencies actually are turning into stuttering. Early intervention usually keeps children from developing negative emotional and social responses to their stuttering. However, just because you are a teenager who stutters, do not think that it is too late to deal with your problem. It is never too late to make some improvement in your speech, even if you are an adult.

Stuttering vs. Disfluency

The diagnosis of stuttering is not easy when children are very young. If you are not sure whether or not you are really a stutterer or simply have a common or mild speech disfluency, consider the following symptoms.

Stutterers have a hard time getting the words out when they want to speak. Their words often "get stuck" in their mouth. Stutterers experience a blocked airflow when they are trying to say a word. A blocked airflow occurs when no air at all comes up through the throat for a couple of seconds. During such a blockage, it is impossible for stutterers to find their voice, and the words they are trying to say simply do not come out. A block may become so intense that the stutterer becomes red in the face, blinks the eyes, and jerks the body around. The physical symptoms of frustration at not being able to speak are obvious.

Stutterers often hesitate before beginning to speak, or they may speak very quickly for fear of stuttering before they finish what they are saying. Once they start talking, they do not want to stop because then they will have to start again, and that makes them nervous.

Stutterers experience distorted physical movements of the muscles that control speech. The muscles affected are found in the lips, tongue, jaw, and soft palate. The soft palate is the soft part of the roof of your mouth between your hard palate, which is right behind your teeth, and your throat. Find it now with your tongue. You can open your mouth wide and look in a mirror to see your hard and soft palates. Stutterers also have a hard time controlling the movements of speech muscles called the vocal folds, located at the back of your mouth near your throat. The vocal folds open and close as you speak to help you form the different sounds that make words understandable. You may be able to feel or see the tension in your face or around your mouth caused by stuttering. You may actually notice that your face contorts (changes into odd shapes) as you struggle to get a word out.

Stutterers have problems with the breathing patterns that are necessary for fluent speech. Rather than breathing evenly, a stutterer's breathing often comes at the "wrong time," when he or she is trying to speak or is already speaking. The pitch and loudness of a stutterer's voice also may rise each time he or she tries to say a word.

Stutterers repeat sounds more than twice, like th-th-th-th-this. A stutterer may repeat a sound more than five times before the actual word comes out. A stutterer may prolong a sound, rather than repeat it, to get through the word, lllllllike this. Stutterers repeat sounds in different places throughout a sentence, not just at the beginning of a sentence. Stutterers may avoid using troublesome words or switch to a different word when they encounter difficulties. They may back up and start a word or thought over again if it did not come out right the first time. Stuttering may come and go, but it is present more often than not. Severe stutterers stutter on more than 10 percent of their speech. Stutterers have good days and bad days, but the stuttering always returns.

Do these speech patterns sound familiar to you? If the symptoms do not sound exactly like your problem, perhaps you actually are just experiencing some normal speech disfluencies. Everyone experiences speech disfluencies at one time or another. You may find your speech becoming disfluent when you are very tired, nervous, scared, or very angry. You may even become disfluent when you are excited and you are having a difficult time expressing yourself exactly the way you want to. But these speech disfluencies pass.

If you still are not sure whether you are a stutterer or someone who simply experiences occasional disfluencies, remember that disfluency involves only the occasional repetition of sounds or syllables. Disfluent speech patterns come and go, and they are more often absent than present.

A person who suffers from disfluent speech often will add "fillers" to his or her sentences, hesitating between words with sounds like "um," "uh," "ah," and "er."

To complicate matters, there are different degrees and patterns of stuttering. You may only stutter occasionally on certain words or during certain social situations, or you may find yourself stuttering almost all of the time, no matter who you are with or where you are. Stuttering can be loosely categorized in three ways: mild, moderate, and severe or confirmed.

Mild Stuttering

Mild stuttering is not much different from normal disfluent speech. The difference is an increase in the frequency and duration of the problem, compared to disfluent speech. This means that the stuttering happens more often and lasts longer. In normal disfluent speech, a person might repeat a syllable once or twice, like this: "Wha-what is that?" A person who stutters will repeat the syllable four or five times, like this: "Wha-wha-wha-wha-what is that?"

The person who stutters also may prolong sounds, like this: "Mmmmmmay I have ssssssome?"

A person's reactions to his or her speech problems can indicate of whether that person is experiencing disfluency or is actually stuttering. A person experiencing a normal disfluency may just laugh it off or say something like, "Gee, I sure can't talk today!" However, a person who is actually stuttering may become upset when he or she stutters. That upset feeling may show itself as eye blinking, blushing, looking off to the side, or tensing of the mouth during stuttering. Another difference between normal disfluency and mild stuttering is that the stuttering will persist. Although mild stuttering may not seem like a big deal to some, if you are the person who is stuttering, it may be a very big deal to you.

Severe Stuttering

Severe stuttering is, of course, much easier to identify than mild stuttering. People who have a severe stutter usually show actual signs of physical struggle when they are attempting to speak. Most severe stutterers will try to hide their stuttering and may even try to avoid talking completely. A person who has a severe stutter will have some disfluency in every phrase or sentence he or she tries to say. These stutters will last for a second or longer. The person with a severe stutter also may show the same physical signs as the mild stutterer, such as blinking the eyes, reddening of the face, looking away or off to the side, and physical tension in facial muscles near the mouth.

The struggle to make words come out also may cause the stutterer's voice to become higher and higher in pitch.

11

Words That Describe Stuttering

As you read through this book, it will be important to understand some of the words used to describe stuttering. Other general words used to describe stuttering are "stammering," "blocking," "repeating," and disfluent speech. You also should be familiar with the terms used to describe exactly what is going on inside of your mouth when you are experiencing the different forms of stuttering. You may not experience all of these types of stuttering, or you may experience some more than others, but it is important for you to be familiar with what is happening when you are having a stuttering spell.

- **Blocking:** Blocking occurs when you try to say a word and the flow of air from your lungs to your mouth completely stops, leaving you unable to make any sound at all.

- **Bouncing:** "Bouncing" is another word for the repetition of sounds and syllables.

↪ **Prolongation:** Prolongation refers to holding on to a sound for a longer period of time than normally necessary, for example, "mmmmmarch."

↪ **Repetitions:** Repetitions are sounds that occur over and over before the complete word is spoken, for example, "ca-ca-ca-ca-can."

↪ **Stuck:** "Stuck" is another word for blocking.

Severe stuttering will be persistent. It will be there almost all of the time, although at some times it may not seem as bad as at other times. However, the stuttering will most likely be with the person every day. Because of this, the severe stutterer may be very frustrated or embarrassed, especially when in a situation in which he or she may be expected to talk to others. On the other hand, even severe stutterers may not stutter when they are singing or whispering or when they are alone or with someone they are very comfortable with.

Moderate stuttering is more frequent and more serious than a mild stutter but less frequent and less of a problem than a severe stutter.

Therapy

Once you know whether or not you actually stutter or simply experience occasional speech disfluencies, you can decide whether or not you need speech therapy. However, it can be somewhat difficult to tell the difference between someone who is showing early signs of stuttering and someone who has a speech disfluency. You can ask your doctor to give you a referral to a speech therapist. The speech therapist will meet with you, evaluate your speech patterns, and help you determine whether or not you are a stutterer. This diagnosis may be a tentative one at first. Your speech therapist may need to meet with you several times to observe your speech patterns before he or she is certain.

Once your speech therapist has decided that you are, in fact, a stutterer, he or she also will be able to determine how severe your problem is and create a therapy plan that is suited to you and your individual needs. For example, someone who has a mild stutter may need only a few sessions of a specific type of word game to produce fluent speech. Someone with a more severe stutter might require more intensive therapy lasting a year or two. Again, do not be worried about this. Your speech therapist will determine what type of therapy you will need and how often you will need it. Your job is to be open and willing to work on your problem. Your success in therapy will depend upon your good attitude.

Stuttering may cause embarrassment and feelings of inadequacy, hurt, fear, shame, and most often frustration. Stuttering, if left uncorrected, may keep a person from enjoying an active social or professional life. So whatever fears you may have about seeing a therapist, it is really a small price to pay for a more fulfilling life. It is not much fun being singled out as a person with a problem, especially a problem over which you seem to have no control. Speech therapists are there to help, not to judge.

Cluttering

There is another speech disorder related to stuttering that should be mentioned. It is not the same disorder as stuttering, but many stutterers also suffer from it. In fact, the symptoms of this disorder often are concealed under the stuttering. This is cluttering. Cluttering is characterized by a rapid or irregular rate of speech, short or long pauses that come in the wrong places, slurring of syllables, and confusing sentence structure. A clutterer does not seem to be certain of what he or she is trying to say, and this person's thought processes seem to start and stop and change direction. A clutterer's speech sounds "jerky" and disconnected, at one moment racing along almost too fast for comprehension, then coming to a halt unexpectedly, and then going off in a new direction.

The clutterer, if he or she is not a stutterer, will not show any signs of stress or frustration when talking, although hyperactivity and sloppy handwriting are symptoms that may be noticed in a clutterer. Treatment for cluttering usually involves teaching a child methods of monitoring and slowing down speech. Most therapy methods designed to help stutterers also will help clutterers, but it is important to diagnose the problem accurately. There may be other learning disabilities present that require different therapy methods.

The Physical
Causes of Stuttering

As you already have learned, stuttering is a speech problem. You also know that doctors and speech pathologists do not yet understand the exact cause of stuttering. They do believe that stuttering is a physical disorder of the nerves and muscles that control speech. Although doctors and speech therapists have not yet discovered the exact cause of stuttering, they have agreed on several things that do not cause stuttering. Stuttering is not an emotional problem. It is not a psychological problem. Stuttering is not caused by something your parents did or did not do to you when you were a child. You need not worry that you stutter because you were mistreated or because you cannot control your emotions. Believe it or not, though you stutter, you are psychologically normal.

Recent research has shown unusual patterns of activity in the right and left halves of the brains of people who stutter. The left hemisphere of the brain, which generally controls speech, shows less than normal activity when someone stutters, and the right hemisphere shows more than normal activity. No one is sure what this means, and in any case, the connection between mental functions and areas of the brain is a very inexact science. We can measure levels of electrical activity in the brain, but we cannot understand thought processes on that level.

Children do not copy stuttering from older brothers or sisters or parents who stutter. Speech therapists have noticed that sometimes children in the same family stutter, and they believe that this indicates a genetic, or inherited, cause. Doctors have not yet been able to prove that stuttering is genetic, but they have done enough research and observation to know that there is a tendency for stuttering to run in families. Whereas the actual stuttering may not be an inherited trait, the susceptibility to becoming a stutterer may be inherited. If you stutter, think about the rest of your family. Does anyone else stutter? Perhaps one of your cousins stutters, or maybe your grandmother stutters. About 50 to 66 percent of all stutterers say that they have a family member who also stutters.

One way that doctors and researchers test their theories about stuttering running in families is by studying twins. When studying identical twins, doctors have discovered that if one twin stutters, there is a much greater chance that the other twin will stutter too. However, when doctors looked at fraternal twins, they found that if one twin stutters it does not mean that the other does. Doctors now believe that stuttering is caused by a combination of hereditary and environmental factors. What this means is that stuttering may run in your family and that your family environment also may contribute to your stuttering. If there are a lot of people in your family, for example, you may find that you must speak quickly to get a word in edgewise; when you speak quickly, you get nervous and tongue-tied, and you stutter. If you are a girl who stutters, you are more likely to have children who stutter than if you are a guy who stutters. This would seem to indicate a genetic cause. However, if stuttering has a hereditary component, exactly what it is is still unknown.

One very important point to remember about stuttering is that it is not something people do on purpose. People who stutter cannot help it, and many are ashamed or embarrassed by their stuttering (although they really should not be, because they cannot help it!). People who stutter are not any different from people who do not, except that they have some trouble making their words come out.

It is difficult to determine the cause of stuttering because there are so few consistent patterns to observe. Although your stuttering probably came on slowly, gradually getting worse and worse over time when you were a little kid, some people start stuttering overnight for no known reason. Some people stutter very badly all the time, and others stutter only a little bit on certain days. The same person can have good days and bad days and can find it almost impossible to figure out why. These patterns puzzle doctors too.

If your stuttering gets worse at times, you may notice that the change occurs in certain situations or when you are nervous, upset, angry, or tired. At these times it becomes even more difficult for you to control your speech muscles, so your stuttering may get worse for a short time. When you are feeling comfortable again, you will notice that you are not stuttering as much anymore. Stuttering is not an emotional or psychological disorder, but your state of mind and your degree of comfort with your surroundings will have an effect on the severity of your stuttering.

Some stutterers say that they stutter more when they first wake up in the morning. Others stutter more when they are trying to speak too quickly. Sometimes stuttering occurs when you are thinking of a word that you want to say, and you know exactly what the word is, but you cannot get that word to come out. You might have noticed that your stuttering gets worse when you try to talk to a particular person—someone in a position of authority, or someone you want to ask out on a date. The nervous tension you feel in situations like this definitely makes you stutter more.

One thing is certain: Even if you stutter a lot, you probably do not stutter all the time. The intermittent nature of this disorder is what makes it so difficult for doctors to study. Stuttering produces some very odd responses that puzzle researchers. You may find that your stutter disappears when you are reading out loud as part of a group. It also has been observed that stutterers do not stutter when they are singing a song! You may discover that you do not stutter when you are talking to animals (your puppy, your cat, your frog). You may not stutter when you are all alone and talking to yourself.

Is It Emotional?

Perhaps you have heard someone say that your stuttering is caused by an emotional problem. Doctors and speech pathologists agree that stuttering is NOT an emotional problem. It is not caused by some emotional trauma you suffered as a child, and you are not an emotionally or mentally unstable person because you stutter. Once again, stuttering is a speech problem, not an emotional problem.

However, there is an emotional component to stuttering. What this means is that although you do not stutter because of an emotional problem, you may have some very strong feelings about your stuttering. Doctors and speech pathologists explain that stuttering has both a psychological and a physical component and that these two components are intertwined. Three factors are involved in the psychological and physical components of your stuttering: your environment; your emotional response to the problem; and the frequency, type, and duration of your stuttering. Let's explore each of these factors.

Environment

Your environment—where, with whom, and how you live—has a great influence on your speech patterns and how you feel when you are talking. Are the people around you calm and patient when you are trying to make your words, or are they hurried and impatient? Do they rush you along when you try to speak and make you stutter even more? Among your family and friends, are you the victim of "verbal bandits" who cut you off before you finish speaking and try to hog the conversation? Having people around you who make you nervous and frustrated when you try to speak creates an unhealthy environment. Trying to speak too quickly does not help a stutterer to speak more fluently.

Emotional Response

How do you react to yourself when you are stuttering? Do you proceed calmly as you try to make your words, or do you get upset and irritated when you cannot get the words to come out right away? Or do you simply refuse to speak unless it is absolutely necessary? Your response to your stuttering is likely to become a habit, so it is important to get it under control. If you let your stuttering bother you on one occasion, you may repeat that response the next time you are in a similar situation. You will experience a never ending cycle of stuttering followed by anxiety followed by even worse stuttering. If you can accept the fact that you stutter and proceed with your life, you will have a much healthier response to your stuttering and will probably stutter less. If you let your stuttering stop you from doing what you want to do or if you let it embarrass you, make you feel ashamed, or hold you back, you are allowing your stutter to have an unhealthy effect on your life.

Frequency, Type, and Duration of Stutter

Your stuttering patterns, that is, how often you stutter, and how long it takes you to get your stuttering under control once it starts, will affect your feelings about your speech problem. You may be a mild, moderate, or severe stutterer, and obviously your frustration will be greater the more severe your problem is. However, there are instances in which someone with a severe stutter may show less anxiety than another person who is only a mild stutterer. The difference lies in personal attitudes of self-worth and how thoroughly someone has accepted the reality of his or her stuttering.

Stress and Fatigue

Stress is part of your everyday life, just like eating and breathing and sleeping. Life without stress is impossible, although it would certainly be nice. Sometimes a stressful situation can become a learning situation. Some people even say that they work better under stress. For example, you may have found that you did a much better job on your science fair project by leaving it to the last minute. Why? The stress of having to get it done in a short time pushed you to put your all into it, and in the end you turned in a great project. However, too much stress, too often, is not good for anyone. Stress is especially bad for stutterers. Although it is known that stress alone does not cause stuttering, stress can cause you to worry about stuttering and thus cause you to stutter even more.

Similar to the effects of stress are the effects of fatigue, or being tired. Again, simply being tired is not enough to make a person stutter, but it does not help. When a person is tired, it is very hard to do anything well, from driving a car to speaking fluently. Just like stress, you can try to minimize your fatigue, but you cannot get rid of fatigue altogether. So accept the fact that when you are under stress or when you are fatigued, you are less likely to have fluent speech.

Fluctuations

Why do you stutter more at some times and less at other times? There is no clear-cut answer to this question. However, some theories exist about why your stuttering seems to "come and go" at different times or in different situations, or why one day you may find yourself stuttering much less than you did the day before. As you have just read, stress and fatigue can play significant roles in when and how often you stutter. Another factor may be the particular person you are talking to. Does this person make you feel comfortable when you speak, or does he or she make you feel uncomfortable? How fast you try to talk also may determine whether or not you stutter more or less. In addition, how you react to particular situations in which you find yourself plays a significant role in how much you stutter. One thing is certain—and most likely you already know this—your stuttering will fluctuate. You will stutter more at certain times than at others.

Childhood Influences

The emotional reaction you and others had toward your stuttering when you were a child may have a lot of influence over how you feel about your stuttering now as a teenager. Consider the following two scenarios:

When Charles was a child and he began to stutter, his brothers reacted poorly. "Spit it out, stupid," his brother Andrew would say. "What's the matter ,Charles? Can't you talk, little baby?" his brother Daniel would tease. "Just say it already, dummy!" his brothers would say when he was having a hard time getting his words out.

Justyna started stuttering when she was very young. Her brother Mike would sit quietly while Justyna worked on getting her words out. "That sounds like fun," he would say when Justyna would tell him about something she had done that day. "Hey, let's go play," Mike would say, being sure to include his little sister in his games so that she wouldn't feel left out.

Who do you think turned out to be better able to cope with stuttering as a teenager? If you said Justyna, you are right. Charles's brothers were mean and teased him as a child, and Charles grew up feeling stupid because he stuttered. He has a difficult time talking to people because he is still afraid that he will be made fun of because he stutters. Charles's brothers did a lot to destroy his self-esteem. He has a hard time meeting new people and making friends, and he does not feel very good about himself. Justyna, on the other hand, was not treated differently by her brother because of her stutter. He spoke to Justyna the same way he talked to everyone else. He had a polite, engaging, and supportive manner. Justyna never felt bad about her stuttering, and in time she grew to have many supportive friends who like her, care about her, and have fun when they are with her. The fact that she stutters does not bother Justyna very much, nor does it bother her friends. Her self-esteem is intact, and she is popular and a good student.

How a stutterer is treated as a child may contribute to how he or she feels about the problem as a teenager. A child who has a mild speech disfluency may outgrow the problem. But if he or she is constantly teased or made to feel upset because of the disfluency, it could become a greater problem. It is important to remember that when you are speaking to a child or even to an older person who stutters, patience and kindness go a long way. If you stutter, you should not determine your self-worth by how you speak. Many important people stutter. Stuttering does not make a person bad, unattractive, or stupid.

Do you remember when you first started stuttering? Do you remember how people reacted to your speech at the time? Perhaps your mother told you to slow down, or your teacher impatiently asked you to speed it up. How did that make you feel? Were you nervous? Annoyed? Embarrassed? Frustrated? If someone made you feel bad because you stuttered as a child, you still may feel bad about your stuttering now. This is a pretty normal reaction. You may be just starting to understand the emotional component of your stuttering, and you may learn that certain circumstances or situations exist that can make you feel uncomfortable. Consider Jill's observation of her brother Max.

"Max hates standing in lines," says Jill. "I don't know why, really, but I think it may have to do with the lunchroom lady at our old school. She was always in a hurry to rush us through the line because there were so many kids who had to get their lunches in a short amount of time. I remember one time when Max was in about fourth grade and the lunchroom lady asked him what he wanted, and Max got nervous and started to stutter.

"'Th-th-th-the p-p-p-p—' Max tried to say.

"The lunchroom lady was impatient and didn't want to wait for Max to get his words out.

"She looked at him and said, 'Spit it out, kid,' which made Max more upset, so he really couldn't speak. Finally she just barked, 'You're getting the meatloaf!' And she plopped a gray slab of meatloaf onto Max's tray. Max looked at me with tears in his eyes when we sat down. 'I h-h-h-hate meatloaf,' he said. I shared my slice of pizza with him, and from then on Max always told me what he wanted, and I ordered it for him.

"Max still hates having to stand in line to order anything. Last week a bunch of us went to the movies, and Max gave me his money and asked me to buy his ticket for him. Then he stepped out of line and waited for us by the entrance. Standing in line makes Max nervous, and it always makes his stuttering worse.

Some people associate their stuttering with a certain event, like Max's experience in the lunch line. Because they had one bad stuttering experience, they expect to have the same problem every time they are in a similar situation. They get anxious and nervous, and consequently they actually do develop the same problem again. They may try to avoid whatever situation makes them feel uncomfortable, the way Max either avoids standing in line or asks someone to place his order for him.

Others stutter only when they are talking to certain people. Max has a problem making requests of strangers, but he does not stutter when he asks Jill to order his lunch or his movie ticket. Max is comfortable speaking to his sister Jill because she already knows that he stutters and does not demand that he speak faster. Jill is patient and waits for Max to form his words and express himself. This helps Max to relax, and he has a much easier time speaking to her than he does speaking to someone he does not know well. You have probably noticed the same patterns when talking to different people.

Stuttering and School

The years you spend in junior high and high school are supposed to be full of fun and excitement as well as quite a bit of self-discovery, learning, growing, and changing. These years can also be fraught with stress and disappointment in addition to some anguish about all the things that are happening as you change from a child to a young adult. Both happy times and difficult times are very normal for teens. As you grow and mature, you begin to discover the characteristics that define who you are as a person, and you also start to develop new interests. You may start to take an interest in your appearance, going parties, magazines and music, and of course, the opposite sex. It is quite a time for you. Life often may be a lot of fun, but sometimes you will find that being a teenager can be more difficult than you expected it to be.

If you are a teenager who stutters, sometimes things may get really difficult for you. Your peers, the other kids you go to school with, may have been very accepting of your stutter in the past, and this is good. But what happens if they suddenly stop being so nice to you, or if you meet new people who don't know you? How do you handle this new situation? How about dealing with dating? Most kids are nervous enough about dating. If you have to worry about your stutter on top of everything else, you simply may decide to avoid dating altogether just so that you do not have to deal with stuttering on a date. Do you see a bad pattern emerging here? You could be letting your stutter get in the way of lots of regular teenage things, and this could be very disappointing, not to mention damaging, for you. So what can you do about it? What can you do to cope with all the new pressures of junior high school and high school as well as stuttering?

You probably spend more time at school and with your friends than anyplace else. Being able to express yourself properly will most likely determine whether or not you succeed in high school. How you speak may determine how well you do in certain classes, especially those in which you are required to answer questions out loud or give oral reports. Your grade in such classes actually may depend on your ability to speak well in front of the class. How you speak also may affect your ability to make friends. If you tend to avoid speaking to other people so as not to stutter, the other kids may think that you don't talk to them because you are either stuck-up, rude, or shy. They may not realize that you are afraid to talk for fear that they may not like you because you stutter. Kids are not always perceptive enough to think that maybe you have a real reason for not wanting to talk. Of course, once in a while you will find someone who is bold enough to come up to you and start a conversation. If this happens, try to look the other person in the eye and simply have a conversation. If you start to stutter, excuse yourself by politely saying something like, "I stutter, but please don't let it bother you." It is almost always a mistake to hide your stuttering.

28

If you are too shy to speak to other kids at school and they do not try to initiate conversations and friendships with you, your high school years could end up being a lonely and less-than-positive experience. But they don't have to be. You don't have to let your stutter ruin this exciting time in your life; you can learn to cope with your it. Participating in your own high school experience is very important if you want to get all you can out of these years, both academically and socially. A few areas may be of particular interest to you, including talking in class, dealing with your teachers, and dealing with your fellow classmates. Let's look at each of these situations separately.

Talking in Class

What is your usual reaction when your teachers call on you to answer a question in class? Do you find that it is easier just to say "I don't know" than to try to answer the question and risk stuttering, even if you actually do know the answer? It is true that by answering "I don't know," you can make your fear of stuttering go away. However, your fear is most likely to be replaced by other feelings of frustration and disappointment that you could not show your teacher that you knew the answer to the question. You may feel annoyance with yourself for stuttering in the first place or a deeper fear that you may never be able to really show people who you are and what you can do.

You will face another difficult and anxious time when your teacher asks you to read out loud. Many teachers call on their students at random to read passages from the textbook in front of the class. By picking students at random, your teacher may make it difficult for you to anticipate your turn and prepare yourself to read. The waiting itself may cause anxiety and increase the likelihood that you will stutter. Other teachers have their students read in the order that they are sitting, or they assign sections to each student before the reading starts. In these cases, you may be able to look ahead to the section that you think you will be reading and study it. You can familiarize yourself with the text and check for difficult words. You can look for any words that usually cause you to stutter.

Unfortunately, you cannot really practice your reading assignment. You will just have to read when it is your turn, and this can be a scary feeling. You may be afraid of stuttering or blocking, and you also may be afraid that your classmates will start to snicker or laugh at you. You may worry that the other students will be uncomfortable listening to you speak when you are stuttering. You might have experienced these feelings on a previous occasion when you read out loud in class. It is normal for you to worry that the same thing will happen again. And what happens when you get nervous or worried about stuttering? You know the answer to that question: You stutter even more!

You also may worry about talking in class when you have to give an oral report. Of course, this is one situation in which you can give yourself a certain advantage. Once you have prepared your oral report, you can practice it by yourself in your room and then in front of your family or some of your friends in order to get comfortable with the words that you are going to use. You will figure out in advance where your trouble spots are, and you can work through them before you actually have to present the oral report in front of your teacher and your whole class. Giving yourself this extra time will give you confidence. If you can give your report with minimal stuttering, you will feel great. The next time you do an oral presentation, you may remember how well you did the last time, and you will have more self-confidence.

Another thing you can do is to ask your teacher if you can have a little extra time during the report and the discussion of your report. If you do not feel pressured to get everything done quickly, you will be better able to relax, ,and you will be less likely to stutter. If you do not have to rush, you will remember to take pauses and breathe properly when you are speaking.

You can try to carry these techniques over to your regular class participation. When a class discussion is going on, you may feel that you ought to keep quiet and not take part, even if you have something valuable to contribute, but how do you feel when you simply sit silently while a class discussion goes on around you? You probably get very bored. How interesting can it be to sit and listen to a discussion and not participate, especially when you have something to say? Imagine getting so frustrated that you end up tuning out the entire discussion, and instead of participating with the rest of your class, you spend your time doodling in your notebook. You can see that this can lead to problems in school. However, if you remember that there is no rush for you to say all the words at once, and if you take the time to express your thoughts slowly and clearly, you will find that participating in a class discussion can be quite rewarding.

For extra help in this situation, speak with your teachers ahead of time, outside of class. Explain to them that sometimes it takes you a little longer to express yourself fluently because you stutter. If they can assist you in keeping other students from finishing your sentences or from cutting you off to say something themselves, you will be a willing and able participant in their class discussions. It is important to share information about your stutter with your teachers. After all, your teachers are there to help you fulfill your potential and get as much as you can out of their class. If you can make them understand your particular needs, you will help them to help you.

Your teachers most likely will appreciate your willingness to discuss your stutter. Most teachers will be very happy to help you cope with your stutter in the classroom. This is not a suggestion to ask your teachers not to call on you in class. If you were to do that, soon you would find that you feel awkward being the only kid in your class who was not required to answer questions or recite out loud. This would make you feel different, insecure, and generally uncomfortable. You stutter, yes, but you are not weird or stupid, and there is no reason why you should allow your teachers to treat you any differently than the rest of the students. Furthermore, if you are never expected to speak aloud in class, you will never get any practice at it, and you will never become confident enough to try it. Go ahead and talk in class. You will feel better about trying than you will if you sit silently. The truth is, you have to talk. You simply cannot get through life without talking!

Once you are in speech therapy, you can work with your therapist on some techniques for talking in class. You may even want to have a conference with both your teacher and your speech therapist to come up with a plan for comfortable classroom speaking. Most teachers will not have much knowledge about stuttering or how to help you, and some of the things they do might not be very helpful at all. A conference with a speech therapist will help.

Your Teachers

Very few teachers come into the classroom with the experience to help students who stutter or to even recognize when a student may be developing a speech problem. In preschool or kindergarten, where many children show speech disfluencies as they are learning to talk, it may be difficult to recognize the appearance of true stuttering. If a teacher is concerned, he or she should not single out a student for special attention. Making a child first aware of a stuttering problem can be emotionally damaging to that child. This initiates the whole process of self-consciousness and anxiety that makes the problem worse. The first step a teacher should take is talking to the child's parents and, if there is one, the school's speech therapist. The student then can be professionally evaluated. For the most part, if a teacher speaks to a student in a calm and patient manner, the child will have fewer problems talking. If the problem is only one of speech disfluency, this calm and unemotional way of talking will help the child to achieve normal speech fairly quickly. The last thing a teacher should do is push a student to talk faster.

With older children, patterns of true stuttering are more evident. The student will show obvious signs of tension and frustration in speaking. Such students need professional help. In the classroom, a teacher can use certain strategies to make things easier on a student who stutters. A lot depends on the attitude of the student. Some children do not seem to be concerned about their stuttering and participate in class normally. Others refuse to talk at all. It is a good idea for teachers to have a private conference with the child to learn a little bit about what kind of person he or she is and to assure the child that stuttering does not bother them. It is important for teachers to give assurances that making mistakes, in speech as in anything else, is normal.

Until the student is comfortable in class or has made progress in speech therapy, there are several things a teacher can do to help. When calling on the student to answer questions in class, a teacher can ask questions that can be answered with only a few words. If every student in class must give an answer, teachers should call on the student who stutters at the beginning, remembering that this student will become more nervous the longer he or she has to wait to speak. Teachers can remind the entire class that they should take their time and answer thoughtfully and that a correct answer, not a quick answer, is the important thing. This will lessen the stutterer's anxiety without singling him or her out. Stutterers have less difficulty when they are reading in unison, that is, along with another person. Teachers can ask their students to read in pairs. With these methods, over time, a stutterer will feel more comfortable in class and may become confident enough to speak on his or her own more often.

It is also important to try to prevent other students from teasing a stutterer. It usually does not help very much to punish students who tease, but teachers can talk to them privately and let them know that tolerant behavior is expected of them. Most children want the approval of their teachers and will respond to such an appeal. Again, using a positive approach, teachers must discourage other students from interrupting someone who stutters. Of course, teachers should never interrupt a stutterer or show the stutterer annoyance or irritation.

Your Fellow Students

If you are very lucky, your fellow students will comprise a group of people who are reasonably mature and understanding, and you will not have to worry too much about their reaction to your stutter. Unfortunately, however, you probably will have some problems with the less mature kids in your school because of your speech problem. Kids, particularly teens, many of whom are very insecure themselves, can be less than tolerant of other people's differences. Some may take out their own feelings of insecurity on the other kids in school. These kids actually look for faults in other people because they think that it will make them feel better about themselves. By cutting others down, they think that they can build themselves up.

This is not a very nice way to act toward other people, as you surely know, but think about it for a moment. Even though you know better, you yourself may have treated another schoolmate this way. Perhaps you teased someone for being the shortest kid in the class, or maybe it was the overweight classmate whom you made fun of. Did you come to realize that what you were doing to this other student is the very same thing that hurts so much when it is done to you? If you came to this conclusion on your own, you should be pleased with yourself and your level of maturity. It is not always easy to admit that you are not being nice or that you are in fact taking out your anger and frustrations about yourself on someone else who actually has nothing to do with your problems.

So what can you do about how other students react to your stutter? You can talk to them. Bring up the fact that you stutter before they have a chance to notice it first and become uncomfortable or make fun of it. Again, this may seem like a stretch for you. You may be used to trying to ignore your stutter, convincing yourself that if you do not acknowledge your stutter, it does not exist. However, to help yourself, you are going to have to confront your stutter and share the fact of it with others. After all, most problems, when brought out into the open, usually are not as big or difficult as they may seem when you are keeping them to yourself.

Carly had always seemed so shy and insecure to Lauren and her friends. They would catch her watching them at lunch, and it seemed as though she wanted to join them but was afraid to ask.

One day Lauren and her friends approached Carly and asked her if she would like to join them at lunch.

"I-I-I-I," Carly began. She was nervous about being approached by them, so she stuttered. Embarrassed, she turned and walked away.

"My friends thought that Carly was being very rude

and that the least she could have done was talk to us. Some of the girls thought she was a snob, and one of them actually called her a pretty mean name."

Carly thought about what had happened and about how much she would have liked to have lunch with Lauren and her friends, and a few days later she approached Lauren when she was by herself.

"I wanted to tell you wh-wh-wh-why I seemed rude the other d-d-d-d-day," Carly began. She looked Lauren right in the eye and confidently said, "I stutter. And sometimes that makes me feel vvvvvvvery embarrassed. I didn't know if you would want me to join you for llllllllllunch if you knew."

Lauren's reaction surprised Carly. She just laughed and said, "Is that all? Well, Megan was sure you thought that you were too good to eat lunch with us!"

Carly laughed at that. "No, I don't think that. I would love to eat lunch with you and your friends."

Lauren introduced Carly to the others. Carly told them, "Sometimes I stutter, but don't worry about it."

"Well, it won't bother us if it doesn't bother you!" Megan said.

Carly felt quite comfortable with Lauren and Megan and their friends after that. The fact that Carly stuttered was almost never noticed by the others once they got to know her. As Carly grew more comfortable with her new group of friends, she actually began to stutter less.

By being up front with Lauren and Megan, Carly was able to help both herself and them. She found out that the girls were much more bothered when Carly seemed not to want to talk to them than by the fact that she stuttered. Often when you tell people that you stutter, you may be surprised to find out how interested they are in it and in stuttering in general. People are often afraid of what they do not understand well. Once you open the door and encourage others to talk about stuttering, you may find that people are not only supportive but quite interested in learning more about the problem and what they can do to help you feel more comfortable when you talk to them.

If you are having an difficult time dealing with a particular group of students, you will find that you will get much further with them simply by telling them that you stutter. Let them see that your stutter does not take away your self-confidence. Once they see that you do not have a problem with your stutter, they will have no ammunition with which to tease you.

You will be amazed at how your straightforward attitude about your stutter will tell people that you will not be treated differently because of it. It is your responsibility to help your friends and classmates feel comfortable with your stutter. The best way to do that is to be honest about it and to show that you yourself are comfortable with it. You can tell your friends about the speech therapy that you attend, and you also may want to comment on your stutter right when it happens. For example, if you stutter on a word, you may want to say something like, "Wow, I just blocked that word. OK, let me see if I can do that better this time."

Another great idea is an oral report! Yes, you can use the occasion of giving an oral report as an opportunity to introduce your classmates and teachers to the fact that you stutter. How? By doing your report on stuttering!

Friends

Is explaining your stuttering to your friends the same as dealing with the kids in your class? Well, not really. Although the two groups may overlap to some degree, your comfort level around your friends is much greater than when you are with your classmates. Your friends know you much better than your classmates do. They have spent much more time with you in far more intimate settings, such as conversations, sleepovers, parties, and family gatherings, than your classmates have. You friends know you the person, not you the person in class who stutters. Your friends may accept your stutter far more easily than someone who does not know you well. However, your friends may do some things that can actually hurt you.

Your friends are the people with whom you share your confidences. You may share your hopes, your disappointments, and your secret crushes with them. You may talk to them about what you want to do or the things that you hate. You may seek the advice of your friends when you are in a sticky situation. You respect your friends' thoughts and opinions, and they respect yours as well. Your friends are there when you need them the most. However, what happens if your friends try too hard to help? Sometimes in trying to help you, your friends may actually be hurting you, and this may happen without anyone realizing it. For example, do your friends ever try to protect you? Protection comes in different forms. Some forms of protection are good, but others are not.

Your friends may try to protect you by not letting you know how they feel about your stutter. They may be embarrassed by it, or they may feel bad for you. Because they feel this way, they may think that it is necessary to do your talking for you. They may talk to your other friends for you, they may talk for you at school or in public, or they may even talk for you around your family. They do this so that you can avoid stuttering and they will not have to feel bad for you. They honestly think that it helps you if you do not have to talk.

Are you in the habit of allowing your friends to protect you in this way? Do you simply say "Me, too" when your friend orders a cheeseburger and fries, instead of saying "I would like a hamburger, medium well, with grilled onions and a side of cheese fries"? It's natural to be nervous in situations like these. You may think that you have to order your food quickly and that the waitress is not going to allow you the time to give your order properly. You can learn in speech therapy how to resist the urge to speak quickly and how to improve your speech fluency so that you can place your own orders and do other things that require you to talk. Depending on your friends to help you avoid these daily problems will only make you more uncomfortable with speaking and increase your frustration.

It may not be easy to tell your friends not to help you out by talking for you, but you need to tell them this, in a nice way if you can. You may worry that you are taking a risk and possibly hurting their feelings, but you have to do what is, in the long run, the best thing for you. Your friends need to understand this. Thank them for showing that they care about you but explain that although they mean well, they really are keeping you from being independent.

New Friends

Have you had trouble making new friends? Do you think that this might be because of your stutter? Some kids are naturally shy and have a hard time starting new relationships. If you stutter, you may feel that your stuttering will make a big difference to people who are deciding whether or not to become friends with you. Stuttering does not need to be an obstacle to new friendships. Your stuttering is a part of you, but it is not the whole person. You have many other positive qualities to bring to a friendship. Think about the things that interest you and that you enjoy doing, and focus on those things rather than on your stutter when you try to establish a friendship with someone. For example, are you a good basketball player? Do you love to ice-skate? Are you really good at math? Do you spend every weekend at the movies? What are the things that make you who you are? Start a conversation with someone waiting in line to get tickets to a concert that you also want to attend. Talk to someone at school who plays the same sports that you play. Join the chess club if chess is your favorite game. You should talk to people about the things that you might have in common with them. This will take the focus of the conversation away from your stuttering.

The best way to handle any of these situations is to talk with your friends in a straightforward manner. Let your new friends know right away that you stutter, in order to put yourself and everyone else at ease.

"I'll Get It!"

This is a common phrase heard around many homes when the telephone rings. If you stutter, however, these may be words that you have never had the urge to say. Talking on the phone is simply a matter of personal preference. Some people absolutely love talking on the phone and can do so for hours on end. Other people prefer to talk in person, write a letter, or send e-mail. Some people just do not like the telephone as a form of communication, whereas others are nervous or afraid of speaking on the phone. Whatever the reasons, it may be of some comfort to you to know that people who stutter are not the only ones who avoid speaking on the telephone.

There is no reason, however, why you should have to avoid the telephone because of your stutter. You can work on your skills with the phone until you become comfortable using it. Start by practicing talking on the phone in a room where you have some privacy or when no one else is at home. Call up a friend or family member who already knows that you stutter and is comfortable with it. You may want to arrange this phone call ahead of time. You can ask your best friend at school if you can call at a certain time in the afternoon. You can tell your uncle or grandmother the next time you see him or her that you would like to call on the weekend. If you cannot prearrange a telephone call, just choose someone whom you feel comfortable calling. Before you start talking, think about what you are going to say. Do not think about the fact that you might stutter. You are still nervous, so this is bound to happen. Eventually you will be able to control your stutter on the telephone. You just need to practice a lot until you are comfortable communicating this way.

You should confront your fears of using the telephone, and you should not try to avoid using it. It is better to stutter on the telephone than to avoid making calls. Speak slowly and softly and don't try to force the words out. If you stutter, that's OK. You cannot always control your stuttering, but you can ease the fear and anxiety that you feel when talking, and your telephone conversations will become easier.

Is It Just Me?

Being a teenager sometimes can mean lonely times, even though you may have a lot of friends and may date occasionally. Even the most popular teens sometimes find themselves at home watching television on a Saturday night. This is normal, but if you stutter, you may think that you are the only teen who ever stays home on a weekend. This is not so. The fact that you stutter may be part of the problem, but certainly it is not the only reason.

If you stutter, you may not be big on talking. If you don't talk, you may not have much chance to make conversation with other kids your age. If you have not been able to develop a few good social relationships, you may find that you do not have a lot of people to hang out with. But this is a situation that you can change. As you develop more fluent speech through speech therapy, you will become more confident in yourself and in your ability to sustain conversations with other people your age. Again, remember that when you do speak to new people, they may be surprised by your stutter. In a positive manner, acknowledge the fact that you stutter, and then relax and allow other people to see that you are comfortable with your stutter. Once they see this, they will relax as well.

Deceiving Yourself

How have you learned to cope with your stuttering up to this point? Do you try to hide it or pretend that it does not exist? Do you avoid talking as much as possible? Do you avoid social situations? Many people try to hide things about themselves that they are not happy with or that they think other people will not like. Someone who hates brown hair might bleach her hair blond, or someone who has bad acne might grow a beard to hide the scarring. There are lots of ways people hide what they consider to be their imperfections: make up, toupees, padded bras, high heels, jewelry, and oversized clothing, to name just a few.

It is not uncommon for people who stutter to try to hide their stuttering from others. If you are spending a lot of time avoiding various activities so as not to be caught stuttering, you are spending too much time worrying about your stuttering. You are letting your stutter take control of your life. Let's look at some of the ways that stutterers hide their speech problem. See for yourself if you are doing any of these things:

↪ Do you generally avoid talking to other people?

↪ Do you avoid participating in group activities?

↪ Do you pretend that you don't know the answers to avoid answering questions in class?

↪ Do you dread meeting new people?

↪ Do you avoid situations that you think would probably be a lot of fun if you did not have to worry about stuttering?

↪ Do you spend time plotting or planning different ways to avoid talking to other people?

↪ Do you feel afraid to ask someone out on a date for fear of stuttering?

↪ Do you let others answer the phone instead of answering it yourself?

↪ Do you sometimes order food from a menu because you are comfortable pronouncing its name rather than ordering what you really want?

↪ Do you wander around in a store trying to find what you are looking for yourself rather than asking a salesperson for help?

➥ Do you often pretend to agree with other people because you are fearful of stuttering through a disagreement?

You may only just now be realizing all the things you have been avoiding because you stutter. Even if only some of these behavior patterns are present, you still are letting your stutter get in the way of many normal activities that should be part of your everyday life. The fact that you do these things may have caused you to experience negative feelings toward yourself. Look at the next list and see if you have any of the following negative feelings:

➥ I stutter because I am stupid.

➥ I stutter because I am nervous. If I could just relax, I wouldn't stutter so much.

➥ I stutter because I am insecure. If I had more self-confidence, I wouldn't stutter.

➥ If only people would not act so impatient when I am talking, I would not stutter.

➥ If I could keep from panicking, I would not stutter.

➥ If I concentrate harder, I will not stutter.

➥ I stutter because I am weak.

➥ If only I just felt better about myself, I would not stutter.

It is fairly normal to have these kinds of thoughts about yourself when you stutter, but surely you can see that thinking this way can be harmful. It is very important not to let your stuttering control who you are, what you do, and how you feel about yourself. Your thoughts reflect the self-doubt and feelings of helplessness brought on by years of stuttering. You probably have tried very hard to stop stuttering, but you have been unable to do so. You may even have developed a worse stutter the harder you tried to stop! That too is a normal experience. Everyone has some self-doubt at some time. Whether it is because you stutter or because you are not happy with something else in your personal life, it is important to recognize that a great deal of self-doubt cannot be anything but self-destructive. The good news is that you really do have the power to change your situation.

I'm in Charge!

One way to begin taking control of your life is to find out all you can about stuttering. This does not mean that you will be able to "cure" yourself or make yourself stop stuttering. There is no cure for stuttering, and it takes a lot of effort working with a trained professional, a speech therapist, to help you control your stuttering. Even if you can figure out on your own why you stutter or under what circumstances your stutter becomes worse, you still will need to seek professional help. However, learning as much as you can about stuttering may help you feel more in control. It may help you to understand exactly what it is that you are doing when you stutter, and why you are doing it. It also may help you to cope with your stuttering in emotional terms.

Once you realize that you can take charge and that you can control your stuttering, you may begin to feel a lot better right away. You must recognize that communication is absolutely necessary in this world and that in order to communicate, you are going to have to talk to people. You already know that when you talk, you stutter. Accepting this fact about yourself will reduce your emotional resistance to talking. It's OK to let people know that you stutter. You can do this in two ways, either by directly saying "I stutter when I speak," or simply by allowing people to discover that you stutter when they hear you talk. You have to decide which of the two options makes you feel more comfortable.

When you take control, you are acting in a mature, responsible way. It is time to move past the point where your parents make all the decisions for you. Of course, as long as you live in your parents' house, they still may have the final say about certain things, and understanding this and being mature enough to accept it is another key part of growing up. However, knowing that you can control your stuttering and that you can control how both you and your friends react to it can be very empowering!

Have you decided that you want to do something about your stutter? If not, that's OK for now. Stuttering may not be the most important thing in your life at this moment. You may change your mind at some point, but even deciding that you do not want to work on the problem now demonstrates that you are taking charge of your life. If you have decided to get professional help for your stuttering, there are a few things that you should remember:

↪ Deciding to work on your stuttering is not enough. You actually have to follow through and work on it.

↪ Doubting that you can change is normal, but don't let doubt get the best of you. You CAN do it!

↪ You will need to make a full commitment to your self-help program. A halfway effort will not help you.

↪ You must work on your stuttering to please yourself, not to please others such as your parents or your friends.

↪ Treatment (speech therapy) for stuttering is not a quick process. It is going to take considerable time and effort, but you will be pleased with the results.

↪ You will have to do the work. No one can do it for you.

↪ Occasionally you may have slight relapses. This is normal. Do not get discouraged.

Telling People
That You Stutter

If you stutter, you may have strong feelings about it. Perhaps you are embarrassed or ashamed.

Take Maryanne's situation, for example. Maryanne is a freshman in high school. She is very interested in acting and has joined the after-school drama club. But she has a problem. When she speaks, she stutters. Her drama coach often asks her to repeat her lines, pick up the pace, and do a better job. All of this makes Maryanne feel very self-conscious about her stuttering. She tends to look away or down at her feet when she starts to stutter. When the stuttering gets to be too much for Maryanne, she says something like, "I forgot what I was going to say, " or "Oh, never mind, it wasn't important." This makes Maryanne even more upset because she feels that people must think that she is a very forgetful or stupid person. Although there is no reason to feel embarrassed or ashamed of the fact that you stutter, you may have experienced negative reactions from other people in the past that make you feel this way.

When it comes to meeting new people, the best way to approach your stuttering is simply to inform the new person that you stutter. When you meet someone new, you can set everyone at ease by first introducing yourself, "Hello, my name is Tyler," and then telling the person that you stutter. "Before we begin to speak, I'd like you to know that I stutter." By letting the new person know what to expect, you will avoid stares, funny looks, or any uncomfortable questions. This new person will not be as likely to try to finish your sentences for you, either. Think about how the following situation might have turned out differently:

> Chris had an interview for a summer job as an assistant in a downtown office. He was nervous about the interview because he was afraid that he might start to stutter and the boss would think he was stupid or incapable of doing a good job. Chris knew that being nervous about stuttering actually could make his stuttering worse. So he tried to calm himself down by slowly repeating his opening line, "Hello, I'm Christopher Thomas." Finally the boss appeared for the interview. Chris stood up and reached for the boss's outstretched hand.
>
> "Good afternoon, I'm Robert Dempsey," the boss said. "Thank you for coming."
>
> "Hello, I'm Christopher Thomas."
>
> "It's nice to meet you, Christopher. Before we begin," said Mr. Dempsey, "I'd like you to know that I occasionally stutter, and I don't want it to make you uncomfortable."
>
> Chris smiled. "Thank you for telling me that, Mr. Dempsey. I'd like you to know that I stutter too."

What if Mr. Dempsey had not told Chris that he stutters? Chris might have told Mr. Dempsey first, which would have been fine. However, if Chris had said nothing, and Mr. Dempsey had stuttered once or twice, and then if Chris also had stuttered, Mr. Dempsey might have become upset, thinking that Chris was making fun of him. The interview then might have gone quite poorly. Mr. Dempsey would have been rather offended, thinking that Chris was being rude and inconsiderate. By clearing the air up front, both Chris and Mr. Dempsey were able to make themselves and each other comfortable. Both Chris and Mr. Dempsey were able to relax, and the interview went quite well.

Your Parents

Your parents know that you stutter. They probably have been listening to you stutter for most of your life. They may be just as frustrated by your stutter as you are. Do they ever talk to you about it? Some parents feel that mentioning your stutter, something that you are very well aware of already, may further upset you or that it may make you think that they are upset with you. Most parents do not want their kids to think that they are disappointed in them. Sometimes parents do not want to bring up the stuttering issue because they feel that it is your private issue and they don't want to intrude. They think that if you really want to talk about it, you will. So in fact, they may be waiting for you to bring it up. Your parents may be trying to respect your feelings. They may not want to embarrass you.

For other parents, the fact that their kids stutter may be no big deal to them at all. They are used to it, and it just would not occur to them to bring it up. In fact, they may be so used to it that they do not even notice your stutter anymore. Or you may be the kind of person who tries to avoid stuttering by talking as little as possible. As a result, your parents may not realize that you still have a problem with stuttering. They may just think that you are a particularly quiet person. This kind of easy acceptance of your problem is both good and bad. On the one hand, you have not been made to feel self-conscious about your stutter. On the other hand, as you begin to confront the world outside your home, your parents' silence on this issue has cut you off from an important source of emotional support.

Another reason that your parents may not talk to you about stuttering is that they really don't know very much about it. They also may feel frustrated that they have been unable to help you control your stuttering. If your parents are not stutterers themselves, they probably have little to share with you in terms of experience, and they have no idea what it is like to be a person who stutters. This may make them feel inadequate and unable to help you.

If you want to talk to your parents about stuttering, you may have to bring the subject up yourself. Most parents will be open to this type of discussion even if they really do not know what it is like to be a person who stutters. They will, nonetheless, want to help you out in the best way that they can. If you share your feelings with your parents, you will not feel so alone, and your parents may have a better time understanding you and your different moods if they understand how much your stuttering bothers you. You have to stop hiding your stutter if you want to get help for your problem. Your parents are the people who care about you the most. Because stuttering is your problem rather than theirs, it is your responsibility to start the conversation with them. This can be somewhat scary. Your first fear, of course, is fear of stuttering when you talk to your parents. To overcome this fear, you simply are going to have to muster up the courage to speak.

You need to find a good place and an appropriate time to talk to your parents. Obviously, trying to talk to them as they are about to go out on Friday night or in the middle of the football game on Sunday afternoon would not be a good choice. A better choice might be at dinnertime or during a long drive. If you don't get much time alone with your parents or if everyone in the family has a hectic schedule, perhaps you should make a formal appointment with them, like Monday night after dinner or Wednesday after Dad's tennis game.

In the beginning, your parents may seem nervous when talking to you about your stuttering. Try to be patient with them. They may be as distressed over your stuttering as you are. They may be afraid that you are going to ask them for advice or answers that they are not equipped to give you. Just remember to be honest and tell it like it is. You can tell them that you are unsure about how to talk about your stutter or that you are feeling embarrassed talking about it, but that you really want to talk. Once you say those words, the rest will come more easily for you. Talk a little bit and then follow up later if that makes you feel more comfortable than unloading everything you feel all at once. One way or another, you have set the stage for discussion, and your parents now know that you are open to talking to them.

Practice Talking to Your Parents

If you are worried about talking to your parents without knowing exactly what you are going to say, you might consider writing your feelings down on paper first. You might write down a few general ideas, or you might write a detailed list of things that you want to discuss. If you are extremely nervous about talking to your parents, you could write out everything you want to say precisely and completely. Putting the words on paper will help you to express yourself exactly as you wish. You can give yourself some extra confidence by practicing what you want to say beforehand in the privacy of your own room. Talk to yourself in the mirror and watch how you look when you are speaking easily and confidently. Say all the words out loud; don't just whisper to yourself.

What to Talk to Your Parents About

Now that you have opened the door to discussing your stutter with your parents, what do you truly want to talk to them about? If you have prepared a list, as previously discussed, what is on your list? You probably will want to start by telling your parents exactly how you feel about your stutter. You may use words like "angry," "embarrassed," or "stupid." Discuss these feelings with them and help them to understand your frustrations. Do they know that you feel this way? Don't forget that it is OK to ask your parents questions, too. Ask them how they feel about the fact that you stutter. And remember that the way your parents feel about your stutter is NOT the same thing as their feelings about you. They may not like the fact that you stutter, but of course they still love you! So do not misinterpret your parents' feelings. You know that you are a good person in spite of your stutter. So do they.

What else do you want to say to them? Talk to your parents about the things that they do that make you uncomfortable. Do they have a habit of finishing your sentences for you? This is a common habit that many parents of teenagers who stutter seem to have. Of course, they are just trying to help you, but it may be very annoying to you, and you should tell them so. More than anything else, your parents have to show patience and allow you to finish what you are trying to say.

You may want to start by explaining to your parents that although they mean well, this kind of "help" really does not help you at all. Explain to them that you become nervous when you have to get all the words out before they say them for you and that this worrying makes you stutter even more. Your parents need to know that you are capable of saying all of your words by yourself. Tell them that the best thing that they can do for you is to be patient, listen, and wait for you to say what you want to say. Ask them to look at the situation from your point of view and to imagine how frustrating it can be when you don't get to finish your own words.

You also can show your parents that finishing your words does not help you. If your parents try to finish your sentences, simply wait for them to finish and then continue with your thought anyway. Finish the sentence for yourself after they have finished the sentence for you. Even if you repeat the same words that your parents have just said, you will demonstrate to them that you are quite capable of speaking for yourself. Your parents cannot stop your stutter, but they can provide understanding and emotional support. In a supportive environment, you will stutter less. If your parents can support your quest for fluent speech, they will be doing you a great service.

You should try to convince your parents not to treat you differently because of your stutter. Some parents seem to understand this instinctively without being told, but other parents need to be reminded. They might not even be aware of what they are doing. Do your parents make excuses for you? Do they tell your friends that you do not talk much because you are shy or because you are the "quiet one"? Sometimes your parents may let you get out of doing things like running errands or making phone calls because they think that it is hard for you to speak to people. Does this make you feel relief and gratitude, or do you feel embarrassed that you are not being asked to do things that other kids your age are asked to do? You must make it clear to your parents that you would prefer to be treated in the same way as your siblings and that you want to be asked to do the same types of things that other teens are expected to do. At first it may be hard for you to run errands and talk to other people, especially if you have been protected from doing so all your life. Have confidence in yourself! You know that you can do it.

There are situations, however, in which a parent's prejudices can be damaging. What if your parents don't think that you need to have speech therapy for your stutter? What if they think that you stutter on purpose or that you could stop stuttering if you really wanted to? Some parents actually think that their teens can stop stuttering if they want to or if they just try harder to speak fluently. Of course, you already know that this is not true, but you need to gently remind your parents of this fact. You stutter because you have a speech disorder. Explain to your parents that no matter how hard you try to prevent it, you stutter anyway, and that sometimes trying not to stutter makes you stutter even more. You should tell them how you have tried to stop stuttering, and you should tell them exactly how you feel—frustrated, scared, tense, or anxious—when you are trying not to stutter. This will help them to understand your feelings and that you are not able to control your stutter the way they may think you can.

If your parents still are not able to understand this, ask your speech therapist to talk to them about this particular issue. Perhaps the therapist will have some words of wisdom for your parents, a way of explaining stuttering in more technical terms than you are able to do yourself. However, what if your parents still do not believe that you need speech therapy? Because they most likely will have to pay for the therapy, their disapproval presents a serious obstacle for you in getting the help that you need. Again, this is a situation in which you have to stand up for yourself and talk to your parents. You should explain to them why you feel that you need speech therapy. You can tell your parents how much the therapy will help you to achieve fluent speech and that you would appreciate their support. If you do not know a speech therapist, you might want to speak with your school counselor or your favorite teacher. He or she might be able to explain your need for speech therapy to your parents. Most school counselors and teachers are not experts on stuttering, but they probably will know enough to understand that this is not a problem you can control and that you need professional help.

If you still are having difficulty getting your parents to understand the nature of your problem, you might want to share this book with them. Showing your parents what the experts have to say may be all it takes to convince them. Furthermore, your parents will be impressed when they realize that you already have taken a step toward solving your own problem by reading this book. Once they see how serious you are, they may be much more willing to accept what you are saying.

Talking to Someone Who Stutters

If you know someone who stutters, you probably are reading this book to try to better understand your friend's problem and to find out how to handle yourself around someone who stutters. Several things are important for you to remember when speaking with a person who stutters:

- ⮫ Do not ask the stutterer to "slow down," "relax," or "take a deep breath." These requests will frustrate the stutterer and possibly cause embarrassment and even more stuttering.

- ⮫ Do not try to finish a stutterer's words or sentences. This may seem helpful, but it will only irritate and frustrate the stutterer more.

- ⮫ Look the person in the eye and act normally. By keeping natural eye contact, you let the person who is stuttering know that it is not making you uncomfortable.

- ⮫ Be patient and wait for the stutterer to get the words out. Your patience will help the stutterer relax, and the words will come more easily.

- ⮫ Speak in a relaxed manner yourself, do not speak so slowly that you insult the stutterer. Speaking in a calm and relaxed manner will put the person at ease and assure him or her that it is not necessary to keep up with your rapid speech.

⇒ Show the person that you are listening to what he or she is saying not how it is being said.

Talking on the telephone with someone who stutters requires patience. People who stutter usually have more trouble talking on the phone than they do talking to someone in person. Perhaps because they feel the need to keep the caller's attention by speaking, stutterers may try to rush their speech on the phone. This does not work well. Trying to speak quickly will make the stutterer falter and have a hard time controlling speech. If you are expecting a phone call from a person who stutters, prepare to be patient and wait for him or her to begin to speak. If you answer the phone and hear nothing, remember that the caller may be a person who stutters and that he or she may be having great difficulty just saying hello.

I Don't Want to Stutter Anymore

By now you have realized that your stuttering is not going to go away on its own, and you probably are wondering if you have to stutter for the rest of your life. The answer is no. Although there is no cure for stuttering, there are many effective therapies to help you learn how to control your stuttering so that you can feel more comfortable when you speak. Most people who get into speech therapy notice a reduction in their stuttering. Some people are able to greatly improve their speech, whereas others are only able to make small improvements. How much your speech improves depends in part on your speech therapist but also on your level of commitment. For a few people, speech therapy is not effective at all. However, this is extremely rare, and there is generally some other underlying problem, such as slow mental development, brain injury, or an unusually strong resistance to the therapy.

Working on Your Own

You might be reluctant to get into speech therapy right away, or you may feel that you can work on your stuttering without help. This may not be the most effective treatment, but it may be a comfortable place for you to start on your journey to fluent speech. If you are reading this book, you probably have already made a few attempts to control your stutter. Did any of these efforts actually help? Probably not. You may have tried to avoid talking too much, or maybe you tried starting all of your sentences with "um" or "uh" in an effort to overcome initial blockages. These techniques might even have seemed to work for you in the beginning, but you soon noticed that they failed to help after a while. You actually may have tried lots of different techniques over the years, and now you are frustrated that none of these things have produced lasting results.

Attitude

Before you become involved in a formal program of speech therapy, you have to realize how important your attitude will be and how hard you will have to apply yourself. As we have said, how you feel about your stutter actually can make it better or worse. If you feel bad about stuttering, you are going to stutter more often. It would be nice if you simply could say "I hate stuttering, so I am not going to do it anymore." Unfortunately, hating your stutter only makes you more conscious of it and more worried about it, and it will get worse. If you can convince yourself that your stutter is not such a big deal, this will actually help you.

How can you convince yourself that your stutter is not a big deal when in reality it has been quite a big deal in your life for many years? First you have to understand the simple truth that everyone has flaws. The old cliche that "nobody is perfect" is perfectly true. The chances are that you are far more bothered by your stutter than the people around you are. In fact, if you are a mild stutterer, people may not notice that you stutter at all. If you are a severe stutterer, people will get used to the way you talk and will not be conscious of your stutter after their initial surprise. A few people may in fact become very uncomfortable with your stutter, but this is their problem, not yours.

Another odd fact is that people are more likely to notice your discomfort about stuttering than your actual stutter. If they seem embarrassed or uneasy, it probably is because they are sensing your own uneasiness. If you can relax, the people you talk to will be more relaxed, which will in turn relax you more. If you can direct your mental focus away from your stutter and stop seeing it as a really huge problem, it won't be! Stuttering should not control you or determine what you do with your life. If you think that people are turned off because you stutter, consider this: Would you be more likely to be turned off by someone who stuttered or by someone who just did not speak to you at all? It is rather difficult to get to know someone who refuses to talk to you! If you feel good about yourself and if you show confidence, this is the image of yourself that other people will see. If you are nervous and embarrassed, other people will pick up on these feelings.

Once you get to know people well, you will not stutter as much when you talk to them. Being close to someone, in a comfortable relationship, reduces your stuttering. And if you know what you are talking about, you also will find yourself stuttering less. Your expertise and knowledge, on the job or when giving an oral report, contribute to your self-confidence. Even if you stutter a little bit, it really is not going to matter that much. Many people who stutter have jobs in which a great deal of talking is required. They have confidence in their ability to do their job well, and they know their material, so they get the job done. All sorts of people, both famous and ordinary, stutter. However, they do not let it get in the way of the life they want to lead. Your attitude toward your stutter, the way you think about it and the way you react to it, will influence not only the way you think of yourself but the way that others think of you too. If you think that you can do something in spite of the fact that you stutter, chances are you can do it!

Developing Confidence in Yourself

Confidence is not something that develops overnight. You need to make a conscious decision to build your self-confidence. On the other hand, try not to have unrealistic expectations, because reaching too far and failing can threaten that growing sense of self-worth. Deal with things at a pace that you are comfortable with and no faster than that. Take small steps. Pause from time to time to take a look at how far you have come. There will be days when you feel as though you have not made any progress at all, and there will even be days when you feel as if you have slipped backward. These are both normal occurrences and nothing for you to get upset about. They are part of the process of working toward your goal. Expect these minor setbacks, accept them, and keep going. You will discover that you actually can build up your own confidence through your failures. You will learn to try, you will fail, and then you will try again and eventually succeed. It will get easier and easier to do this. You will learn from experience and discover better ways of doing things so that you will not fail quite so often.

Whenever you try something new, whether it is ice skating, basketball, or asking someone out on a date, there is a good chance that you will fail. Failure can hurt, sometimes for a long time, and you will feel bad when you don't accomplish what you set out to do. This happens to everyone, not just to people who are trying to control a stutter. However, by making the effort, you will build your self-confidence. The next time, you will know what you did that did not work and what you can do differently for a better outcome. There is always something to be learned from each failure, just as there is something to be learned from each success.

Always bear in mind that your feelings and the way you act are closely tied together. If you feel confident when you speak, you will feel relaxed, and even if you stutter, you still will speak the words that you want to say. Your words will come out because you have the confidence to allow them to. Try this out by acting strong and confident, and you will find that you are strong and confident. Be proud of yourself for the hard work that you are doing, and keep working.

A Self-Examination

What exactly is going on inside your mouth when you try to talk and end up stuttering? It will be well worth your time to study the physical process of stuttering. After all, it is pretty difficult to change something if you don't know exactly what it is that you are doing wrong. It is time to take a look at yourself and your stuttering and find out exactly what it is that you are doing.

You will need to find a quiet place where you can be alone, and you will need a mirror. Look at yourself in the mirror and start talking. It doesn't really matter what you talk about. Put your hand on your throat. Feel the sounds that your throat makes when you talk. Now hold your hand in front of your mouth. Feel your breath flowing as you talk. Stutter. If you cannot force a stutter when you are talking to yourself, pretend. Pay careful attention to how your face, your mouth, your jaw, and your throat change shape and how your breath feels when you are stuttering. Note the differences between stuttering and not stuttering. What are you feeling? Do you feel any tightening of muscles? Are you trying to push your words out? Is part of your speech system simply not doing its job?

Stuttering can take many different forms. You may have problems with certain words or sounds. Other sounds may cause you no problem. See if you can recognize when and how you stutter and when your speech is fluent. Pay close attention to each element of your speech. You should start to get an idea of what is happening when you stutter, which muscles tense up, how your airflow is blocked, and which sounds cause the greatest problems. Armed with this knowledge, you can practice difficult sounds and really feel what is happening inside your mouth. You may be surprised, but your speech probably will improve a bit as a result. The change will begin to happen if you stay focused on doing this exercise patiently.

It is important not to avoid the difficult sounds. If you

avoid trying to sound out the hard words, you will never be able to figure out what your muscles are doing and what sounds you need to work on. In other words, you are going to have to stutter more in order to stutter less. Accept the challenge. You may be surprised to discover that the hard words are not that hard to say once you stop being afraid to say them.

The greatest problem stutterers face is speaking too quickly. You must learn to speak slowly. When you want to say something, don't just rush into it. First think for a moment and begin the words slowly. Do not be afraid of the words, and don't tighten up as you say them. Start each word on one slow sound. Hold the starting sound and then move into the word gradually. You can finish the word at a normal pace, but you need to get through the initial stutter slowly. Try it alone at first, and when you have enough confidence, try speaking in front of others.

This is a good start, but you have probably come to realize that although these techniques produce some improvements, you are going to need extra help. It is time to consider a speech therapist. Although you have been working on helping yourself and you may be getting somewhere with it, you will do even better in speech therapy. Your speech therapist can point you in the right direction and show you which way to focus your energy. A speech therapist will be able to do some things for you that you cannot do for yourself, such as demonstrating vocal techniques and helping you track your progress.

Now is the time to get yourself into speech therapy.

Speech Therapy

So you have gone about as far as you can go on your own, and you are ready for the help of a professional speech therapist. It is important to realize when you are starting speech therapy that there is no quick fix, instant cure, or magic pill to help you control your stuttering. Your goal in therapy will be to develop fluent speech, not to avoid stuttering. The difference between these two goals is a matter of emphasis, but it is important. To avoid stuttering, it is possible to use such techniques as switching words or saying something other than what you really want to say. This may be what you have been doing up to this point, but it is definitely not the goal of speech therapy. The goal of speech therapy is to make you as comfortable and relaxed as possible with your stuttering so that it is minimized. The goal of therapy is to remove the psychological barrier to expressing yourself. Therapy is based upon the idea that it is better to speak and stutter than not to speak at all.

Speech therapy to control your stuttering can take six months to two years of hard work. You probably will have to meet with your speech therapist for one to two hours every week in the beginning, and you will have to do the homework your speech therapist gives you. This may sound like a lot of time and effort, but it's not so long when you think of the alternative: stuttering badly for the rest of your life. If you are wondering why speech therapy is such a long process, remember that you have spoken the way you do for your entire life, and habits can be extremely hard to break or change. Your stuttering problem also may involve deeply felt emotions such as fear, anger, embarrassment, and shame. You will need to work on changing your feelings about your stutter at the same time as you work on your actual stuttering.

Counseling

Counseling is a part of speech therapy. Its purpose is to deal with the feelings you have about your stuttering. Sometimes your speech therapist also can provide you with the emotional counseling you need to overcome your stuttering. If your emotional problems are too great, however, your speech therapist may not feel equipped to deal with them and may refer you to a psychologist, psychiatrist, or social worker. Your counselor is not going to search for the cause of your stuttering in some childhood experience. He or she simply will try to understand you as a person and teach you to have confidence in yourself during the course of therapy. With counseling you will gain a better understanding of how your nervousness and anxiety make your stuttering worse.

Your Speech Therapist and You

How you feel about your speech therapist can have a great impact on how well you do in speech therapy. If you are uncomfortable around your speech therapist, you will have difficulty making progress. If you feel at ease with that person, you are more likely to see improvement in your speech. If you have any bad feelings about your speech therapist, you should choose a new one right away.

When you are choosing a speech therapist, there are some things to keep in mind. The speech therapist at your school may be a pleasant and well-educated person, but unless he or she specializes in stuttering, that person probably will not have the expertise to help you. You would be better off finding a speech therapist through a referral from your family doctor, through a nearby hospital, or by calling the Stuttering Foundation of America for the name of a specialist in the field. The Stuttering Foundation of America provides these referrals for free, and its telephone number can be found in the Where to Go for Help section at the back of this book. One of your concerns should be the amount of time the therapist can devote to working with you one-on-one. You are making a commitment, and you want one from your therapist as well.

Talk to other people who have worked with the speech therapist you are considering. You can ask questions and find out how other patients judged their progress under this particular therapist's care. If the speech therapist is reputable, he or she should not have a problem giving your name to a few patients. Because it is unethical to give out the names and phone numbers of patients without their consent, they will have to call you. Be wary of a speech therapist who gives out personal information about patients. If the speech therapist does provide you with the names and phone numbers of patients, ask these people if they have consented to having this information given out.

When you are looking for a speech therapist, be sure to look for one who has had special training and experience in working with people who stutter. Your therapist should have a Certificate of Clinical Competence from the American Speech-Language-Hearing Association. Here are a few questions you can ask during an interview:

> ↬ How many years of experience do you have working with people who stutter?

> ↬ How many people have you seen altogether in your career as a stuttering specialist, and how many are you working with right now?

> ↬ What is your success rate with those you have worked with?

> ↬ What does your treatment focus on?

You are going to be spending a lot of time, energy, and money with your speech therapist, and it is your right to know all about his or her professional background. If he or she seems uncomfortable or offended by any of your questions, this is probably not the speech therapist for you.

What Will You Learn in Therapy?

The key to controlling your stuttering is learning to speak in smooth, connected phrases as opposed to short, choppy ones. Your speech therapist will introduce you to a number of techniques designed to help you achieve this. You will learn how to:

71

↪ Pause and start slowly when you want to speak.

↪ Cause an easy onset of phonation (slowly initiating the movement of vocal cords to make sounds).

↪ Learn to use a slower rate of speech.

↪ Use light articulatory contact (using light and easy touches of your tongue and lips to make word sounds) to relieve the muscle tension you feel when you are trying to speak.

↪ Make vowel sounds last longer when you say them.

↪ Pause appropriately between words, sentences, and thoughts.

The purpose of these techniques is to help the stutterer achieve a kind of speech that is fluent, but slightly slower than normal. Then the therapist will work with you to make that speech more normal-sounding and to help you to speak faster. You also will practice exercises designed to help you relax your breathing. When people are about to speak, they usually take a quick, large breath, using their upper-chest muscles to expand their lungs. They hold the air in their lungs, exhaling just enough air to sustain speech, and they usually finish speaking before they require another breath. Controlling air flow in this way increases pressure in the lungs and tension in the throat muscles. Muscle tension, of course, is a big problem for stutterers.

Your therapist will teach you a more relaxed way to breathe, using your diaphragm, the muscle inside your lower chest above your stomach. This causes you to take more and smaller breaths and to breathe more gently, lowering the pressure in your lungs and the tension in your throat muscles. As a result, initially you will be able to speak only in short phrases of a few words each before you have to take another breath, but your speech will be more relaxed and fluent.

You may have found that certain sounds are harder for you to say than others, although this varies from person to person. Usually a person who stutters has a harder time with the voiced consonants, such as *d, m, l,* and *r,* and vowels, than with the voiceless consonants such as *t, p,* and *f.* If you listen carefully and feel your throat as you talk, you will observe that voiced consonants involve some vibration of the vocal cords, whereas voiceless consonants do not.

Your speech therapist also will help you to get over your fear of certain words or sounds. There may be a particular sound that you have had a lot of trouble saying in the past. You may have developed the habit of avoiding words that start with that sound. Your speech therapist will help you to feel comfortable saying that sound successfully. Your speech therapist may help also you to get over your fear of certain words that you may have difficulty with. This is called word desensitization.

In addition, your speech therapist can help you to work through any anger you may feel about your stuttering. A good speech therapist will give you a chance to vent your feelings about your speech problem. Talking to someone about your feelings is an important part of your speech therapy. This part may take a few sessions; that is quite all right. Trying to rush your speech therapy most likely will have a negative effect on your progress.

Making Progress

Your speech therapist will teach you to coordinate your speech so that it is fluent. To do this she will start you off slowly, with short, easy exercises. She may have you begin simply by having a conversation with her so that she can evaluate your problem and your specific needs. She may have you read words out loud, one at a time, or passages from a book or a short story in a magazine. After some time she may open the door to your therapy room, and then she may ask another speech therapist to join you in the therapy room. Her purpose is to expose you to a larger and more complex environment as your speech improves. After more therapy, she may have you walk around the therapy facility with her. Perhaps you will walk the halls, visit the gift shop, or stop at the front desk and speak with the receptionist. When your therapist feels that you are ready, she may ask you to repeat these exercises by yourself while she watches you from a distance. Although you may have learned to speak well within the confines of your therapy room, you also have to learn to speak in public situations. By supervising you as you attempt to make your way in a public situation, the therapist is giving you the confidence to go at it on your own.

Speech Therapy and Your Family

Your family's behavior and attitude toward speech therapy may have a strong impact on how well you do. For example, if you depend on your busy mother to drive you to therapy once or twice a week, she sometimes might feel stressed about it, and you may sense her anxiety. This can make it difficult for you to concentrate in your therapy session. It might be easier to take public transportation or to walk to your appointment by yourself. If your parents are rushed when the speech therapist is explaining things, or if they are not supportive of your desire to improve your speech, you may find it difficult to continue.

There are several things you can do if you find yourself in these types of situations. You can ask your parents to be more understanding. You can ask your therapist to speak to your parents about the situation. If your parents seem too busy to take you to therapy appointments, you might ask your therapist if it is possible to conduct sessions at your home. The idea is to make the therapy comfortable and workable for you and everyone around you so that you do not experience the anxiety that slows your progress.

Attitude Is Everything

Therapy of any sort works only if you are committed to it. You will not make progress if you are not willing to work at your speech therapy. Until you are ready to accept your stuttering as a problem and seek help, you will not be a good candidate for speech therapy. If, on the other hand, you have come to terms with the fact that you no longer can handle your stuttering and you are willing to do all it takes to help yourself through therapy, you are ready to become a partner with your speech therapist. If you go into speech therapy with a good attitude, you are much more likely to succeed than if you go in with a poor one.

What Can You Expect?

For some people therapy works quite well, and their stuttering becomes barely noticeable. Others, although they still may stutter noticeably, will be happy with less dramatic results because they *feel* as though they are speaking better. Their self-esteem has improved, and they feel more in control of their speech. If a stutterer feels that he or she is speaking better, the person will begin to relax when talking. The more relaxed you become about your stuttering, the less likely you are to stutter. This is not to imply that stuttering is all in your head, but it is a problem that you can have some control over once you learn how.

In the Session

In the first few sessions of speech therapy, it may seem as if your speech therapist is not doing very much. She simply may ask you questions about school, your friends, or what things are like for you at home. Although this may not seem like speech therapy to you, what your therapist is doing is evaluating you. She is trying to learn about your stutter by talking to you. She will be listening for certain patterns in your speech and deciding how and when you stutter. She will ask you questions about your life to find out if there are certain situations in which you stutter more than others. You need not be concerned with the details of what your speech therapist is doing at this time. If you worry about it too much, you may not be able to give the speech therapist a clear view of your problem. Do not try to second-guess the therapist or give the answers that you think she would like to hear. Just relax and try to get comfortable. It is very important to feel comfortable in your therapy sessions.

Your speech therapist may tape-record your therapy sessions. She will study the tapes after the session to listen for certain speech habits that you may have developed. She also may bring the tapes back into therapy at a later date so that you can listen to the way you spoke in the first sessions and compare your earlier speech to your present speech. This is a good way to measure how far you have progressed after a certain period of time. Do not worry if your speech therapist does not tape your sessions. Each speech therapist will have his or her own individual way of working.

Practice, Practice, Practice

Once you have begun speech therapy, you will need to make a commitment to practice what your speech therapist is teaching you. Practice in your room by yourself. Practice in front of a mirror so that you can see how your mouth, jaw, and face move when you are speaking correctly. When you feel more confident about the progress you are making, practice speaking with your family or close friends. Practice on the telephone, practice in social situations, and practice in public. Practice diligently. You will see the results of your practice, and you will feel a new confidence brought on by your improved speech.

Your Situation Journal

One very effective way for you to explore your own feelings about stuttering is to keep a situation journal. Your speech therapist may ask you to begin a situation journal when you start your speech therapy. In this journal you will write about situations you find yourself in, such as whom you were with, whether or not you had a problem with your stuttering, and how you felt at the time. By keeping this journal, you may find some clues that reveal what triggers your stuttering. You will note the times when your stuttering seemed worse and record how your feelings were reflected in each situation. You will become more aware of what you are doing and how it feels when you are stuttering.

Study this journal after you have built up a fair number of entries. You will discover patterns. You may learn that certain feelings make you stutter more intensely or that stuttering makes you feel a certain way. Pay special attention to situations that involve your teacher, your boss, the telephone, waiting in line, or ordering food—commonly stressful situations for stutterers. For example, Fred discovered that whenever he calls for a pizza, he orders mushrooms and sausage. "I really don't like sausage as much as I like p-p-p-pepperoni," Fred explains, "but whenever I say p-p-p-pepperoni, I stutter. And I don't want to stutter over the phone, so I always order sausage instead." When Fred orders pizza, he unconsciously anticipates the problem he is going to have and chooses a different word. Fred was letting his stuttering get in the way of what he really wanted. By recording these events in his situation journal, he was able to realize what he was doing, and now he is working with his speech therapist on saying the word "pepperoni."

Fear of Failure

One more point about speech therapy should be mentioned here. If you were in speech therapy as a child and you still are stuttering now as a teen, you might think that it will not work for you. You may be afraid to try speech therapy again. However, you will not outgrow your stutter, and you will need speech therapy to work it out. You can talk to other people who have been through speech therapy to find out more about how and why it worked for them. Ask them how they felt before they started it and how they felt once they were in speech therapy. Listen to the way their speech sounds now. Of course, you will not have the exact same experience as others, but by talking to them, you can get some idea of what to expect once you are in therapy.

The Results

A number of factors will affect the results of your speech therapy. One of these is the actual severity of your stuttering. Another factor is your attitude and your willingness to work hard. Your speech therapist's expertise in the field of stuttering is another important factor. Also, your family's ability to support you will play a large part in your progress. Even if not all circumstances are favorable, this does not mean that you are going to fail. It does mean that you may have to work a little harder to achieve your goals. Of course, once you get through all of the hard work and actually reach your goal of fluent speech, you will feel a great deal of pride in yourself and all that you have accomplished.

It will be a great help to you to get started on speech therapy as soon as possible. Even if you did not have the chance to get speech therapy when you were a child, it is not too late to take care of your stuttering now. A late start can cause problems, however. For some kids, stuttering causes them to withdraw from friends and family and even from speaking altogether. If you face your stuttering before you start to hide it or avoid social situations, you will be better off. Whether or not you got help early, the fact that you are getting help now is what really matters.

Remember that there is no cure for stuttering. Beware of any speech therapist who claims to be able to cure you of your stutter. A good speech therapist will tell you that she can help you, but not that she can cure you. You may improve your speech a great deal through speech therapy. You may even think of yourself as "cured" if you are able to achieve a level of fluency that pleases you. What matters is that you are happy with the progress you are making.

Life and Work

To summarize, there is as yet no cure for stuttering, and there are no simple answers for stutterers. Researchers are beginning to zero in on the genetic markers for susceptibility to stuttering, and the future may bring new treatments with drugs and other therapeutic procedures. For now there is no cure. With speech therapy and a lot of hard work, you can reduce your stuttering, but the real purpose of therapy is to make you less nervous and more comfortable when you communicate with people. The more comfortable you are, the less you will stutter. However, you have to accept the fact that you still will continually stutter sometimes for the rest of your life, and you will have to work at making yourself speak without anxiety. This is not to say that you cannot make enormous improvements in your speech fluency. In fact, with hard work, you may reach the point where you are so relaxed about talking that you don't even notice your stutter. Other people may also become so comfortable with you that they do not notice your stutter either. The point is to eliminate stuttering as an obstacle to a normal and fulfilling life.

Work

What about getting a job? Will you experience discrimination in a job interview? Will you be permitted to do the work you like and have been trained to do? Unfortunately, studies have shown that 85 percent of employers believe that stuttering will affect a person's chances of getting a job or a promotion. Other studies have shown that some employers are more comfortable hiring someone who is deaf than someone who stutters. Stuttering is so poorly understood that many employers regard people who stutter as "strange," as somehow different from people who suffer other types of common disabilities. This puts the responsibility on you to tell interviewers and employers of your speech problem and to educate them about it. No one is qualified to do every kind of work. As much as we might want to, most of us cannot be astronauts or championship boxers or rock stars. However, you are qualified to do almost any kind of work that can be done by people who speak fluently, including jobs that require you to talk quite a bit. You should expect to be judged on the full range of your talents and abilities, not by how quickly or smoothly you speak. Even nonstutterers experience some disfluency in about 2 to 4 percent of their speech. And even actors and politicians, whose stock in trade is good public speaking, have overcome stuttering and made successful careers for themselves.

Your Rights

If you believe that you have been discriminated against in a job interview or on the job because of your stutter, what are your rights? As one would expect with the law, the situation is complicated. The Americans with Disabilities Act, passed by Congress in 1990, prohibits discrimination against qualified disabled individuals in job applications, promotions, salaries, job training, and other employment benefits. The act defines a disability as a "physical or mental impairment that substantially limits one or more of the major life activities" of a person. The Equal Employment Opportunity Commission has interpreted this act to cover "any physiological disorder" affecting "speech organs."

This book has argued that there is no reason that stuttering should limit "major life activities," and that stuttering is a "disability" only if you allow it to become one. In another context, the Supreme Court has considered this very issue. In *School Board of Nassau v. Arline,* the Court decided that even if a certain disability did not limit major life activities or the technical ability to perform a job, it could qualify as a disability if a person's work was affected by the prejudices or stereotypes of employers or other employees. The Supreme Court said that "society's myths and fears about disability and disease are as handicapping as are the physical limitations that flow from actual impairments." If you are not hired for a job because your employer believes that other employees will react negatively toward you, and for no other reason, you may be able to prove discrimination under the Americans with Disabilities Act.

A Final Word

Of course, at this point in your life, you are not concerned about lawsuits or confrontations with employers. You just want to get through high school and your teen years with a minimum of discomfort and embarrassment. You want to be accepted by your friends, classmates, and teachers, and you want to be able to communicate with them without anxiety. You want to be able to accept your stuttering, live a normal life, and participate in all the activities you are interested in.

In order to do that, you have to remember that although you stutter, you are a normal teenager. You are intelligent and determined. Your stutter is a problem that you likely will have to cope with for the remainder of your life. However, you do not have to let your stutter get the best of you. You can graduate from high school, go to college, get the job you want, get married, and have children. It's all possible if you have the courage and determination to get the help that you need. Remember how many famous and successful people have managed to overcome their stutter and make big names for themselves. Lawyers, doctors, teachers, and other everyday people enjoy successful, meaningful, and fulfilling lives despite that fact that they are stutterers. If you are determined, you can get through this. Remember all that you have read about confidence and helping yourself. You are at the beginning of a long but very exciting journey of self-discovery and self-fulfillment. You are doing this for yourself, not for anyone else. In the end, you will be the one who benefits the most from all of your effort. It will be your success story.

Glossary

avoidance   A stutterer's attempt not to stutter.

blocking   When the airflow from your lungs to your mouth completely stops, leaving you unable to make any sound at all.

bounce   The unintentional repetition of the first sound or syllable of a word.

easy onset of phonation   Slowly initiating movement of the vocal cords to make sound.

initiating   Starting to speak.

light articulatory contact   Using light and easy touches of your tongue and lips to make word sounds.

phonation   Producing the voiced sound that is speech.

prolongation   Holding a sound longer than usual.

repetition   A sound that is made over and over before a word is completed.

speech therapist/speech pathologist   A person who is professionally trained to treat speech disorders.

speech therapy   Treatment for a speech disorder.

stammering   Another word for stuttering, more commonly used in England.

stuck   Another word for blocking.

word desensitization   Therapy to help you get over your fear of saying words that you stutter on.

Where to Go for Help

The National Center for Stuttering
(800) 221-2483
Web site: http://www.stuttering.com

National Stuttering Project
5100 East La Palma Avenue, Suite 208
Anaheim Hills, CA 92807
(800) 364-1677

Ontario Association of Speech/Language Pathologists and
Audiologists
22 College Street, Suite 300
Toronto, ON M5G 1K2
Canada
(416) 920-3676

Speech Foundation of America
152 Lombardy Road
Memphis, TN 38111

Stuttering Foundation of America
3100 Walnut Grove Road, Suite 603
P.O. Box 11749
Memphis, TN 38111-0749
e-mail: stuttersfa@aol.com
Web site: http://www.stuttersfa.org
(800) 922-9392

For Further Reading

Bobrick, Benson, and Deborah Baker (eds). *Knotted Tongues: Stuttering in History and the Quest for a Cure.* Tokyo: Kodansha International, 1996.

Fraser, Jane, and William H. Perkins, Ph.D., eds. *Do You Stutter? A Guide for Teens.* Memphis, TN: Stuttering Foundation of America, 1992.

Hullit, Lloyd M. *Straight Talk on Stuttering: Information, Encouragement, and Counseling for Stutterers, Caregivers, and Speech-Language Clinicians.* London: Charles C. Thomas Publishers, 1996.

Johnson, Karin L., and Barbara A. Heinze. *Fluency Companion: Strategies for Stuttering Intervention.* East Moline, KS: Linguisystems, 1994.

Rustin, Lena, Robert Spence, and Francis Cook. *Management of Stuttering in Adolescence: A Communication Skills Approach.* San Diego, CA: Singular Publishing Group, 1995.

Schwartz, Martin F. *Stutter No More.* New York: Simon and Schuster, 1991.

Weber, John C. *Coping for Kids Who Stutter.* Vero Beach, CA: The Speech Bin, 1993.

Index

Index

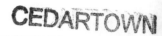